QUICK & EASY HOTPOTS AND STEWS FOR BEGINNERS

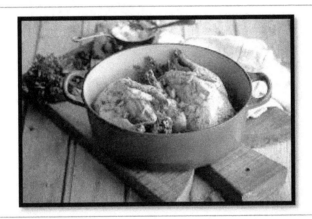

*The Ultimate Beginner's Guide with More than 50
Meal Prep. Learn How to Prepare Delicious Dishes
Quick and Easy, and Build a Complete and Healthy
Meal Plan Made With the Best Flavors of the World
and Mainly of the Mediterranean Diet. This
Cookbook Is Suitable for All the Family*

Isabel Lauren

Welcome

"QUICK & EASY HOTPOTS AND STEWS FOR BEGINNERS" is a cookbook I've realized after collecting the best Stew, Hotpot and Casseruole recipes I tasted in my travels around the world.

I personally love this type of dishes because I find them very tasty and you can do other things while cooking, and you sure make a good impression on your guests!

The reasons to choose Hotpots and Stews of are so many, I want to remind you the most important below.

5 Reasons to eat Hotpots and Stews

1. <u>MANAGE YOUR TIME</u>

Hotpots, Stews and Casseruoles are the best if you want to prepare delicious dishes but you are busy. Infact, with these types of cooking, you can cook dishes saving time, or, better, optimizing time and being able to carry out other activities while cooking.

2. <u>SATISFY GUESTS</u>

Hotpots, Stews and Casseruoles are great dishes to present when you have guests at home. They are very versatile and you can cook many different foods this way, and to satisfy everyone's tastes. What's better than an excellent tasty dish to share with friends during a lunch or dinner?.

3. **SLOW COOKING AT LOW TEMPERATURE**

Hotpots and Stews are based on slow cooking, which allows the heat to spread slowly and constantly and have a better final quality of the food. In the same way, even the low temperature and the stewed cooking ensure that the organoleptic qualities of the meal remain unaltered ultil it is ready to eat.

4. **COOKING WITHOUT CHECKING**

Often the most boring part of cooking is properly having to constantly check the cooking, so that the dish does not burn or cook in a heterogenous way with a final result not perfect. Hotpots will avoid this inconvenient thanks to a slow and homogeneous cooking. Without always having to check and so you will be able to carry out other business in the mean.

5. <u>**SUITABLE FOR MANY FOODS**</u>

With this type of cooking you can prepare many different foods and satisfy the tastes of each person. In fact, you can cook excellent dishes of meat, fish, vegetables at home. legumes and even fruit. Moreover, with Hotpots and Stews you can easily get complete meals in only one pot.

So, what are you waiting for?

Immediately start testing some recipes from the cookbook!
Good fun and if you want, add your personal pinch to my recipes!

Table of Contents

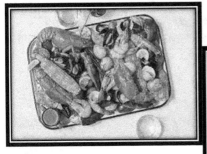

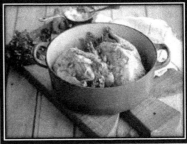

QUICK & EASY
HOTPOTS AND STEWS
FOR BEGINNERS

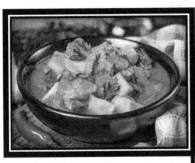

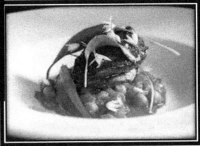

Beef Hotpot

Ingredients:

- 2 lb rump steak, cubed
- 12 oz carrots, thickly sliced
- 2 onions, thickly sliced
- 1,5 lb potatoes, thickly sliced
- 18 fl oz beef stock
- salt
- freshly ground black pepper

Procedure:

1. Preheat the oven to 325°F.
2. Arrange a layer of beef in a casserole dish.

3. Sprinkle over a little salt and pepper, then top with a layer of carrots, onions and potatoes.

4. Pour in the stock.

5. Cover and bake for 2–21,5 hours until the meat is tender.

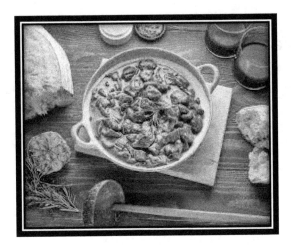

6. Increase the oven temperature to 400°F, and cook for another 30 minutes or until potatoes are brown.

7. Serve hot.

Turkey One-Pot

<u>Serves 4</u>

Ingredients:

- 4 oz dried kidney beans, soaked overnight and drained
- 1 oz butter
- 2 herby pork sausages
- 1 lb turkey casserole meat
- 3 leeks, sliced
- 2 carrots, finely chopped
- 14 oz canned chopped plum tomatoes
- 3 teaspoons tomato purée
- 1 bouquet garni
- 14 fl oz chicken stock
- Salt
- freshly ground black pepper

Procedure:

1. Cook the beans in boiling water for 40 minutes, then drain well.
2. Meanwhile, heat the butter in a flameproof casserole dish, then cook the sausages until browned and the fat runs. Remove and drain on kitchen paper.
3. Stir the turkey into the casserole dish and cook until lightly browned all over, then transfer to a bowl using a slotted spoon.
4. Stir the leeks and carrots into the casserole dish and brown lightly
5. Add the tomatoes and tomato purée, and simmer gently for about 5 minutes.
6. Chop the sausages and return to the casserole dish with the beans, turkey, bouquet garni, stock and seasoning.
7. Cover and cook gently for about 1,25 hours until the beans are tender and there is very little liquid.

Serve hot.

Lamb Hotpot With Dumplings

Serves 4–6

Ingredients:

- 1,5 lb neck of lamb, chopped
- 2 teaspoons redcurrant jelly
- 2 onions, chopped
- 1 pt vegetable stock
- salt
- freshly ground black pepper
- 3 carrots, chopped
- 1 turnip, chopped
- 6 oz mushrooms, sliced
- 1 parsnip, chopped and blanched
- 1 tablespoon tomato purée

For the dumplings

- 4 oz self-raising flour, sifted
- 2 oz suet, shredded
- 1 teaspoon chopped fresh parsley

Procedure:

1. Preheat the oven to 375°F.
2. Put the pieces of meat in the bottom of a large casserole dish. Spread them with the redcurrant jelly, and put in the oven for 15 minutes.
3. Remove and add the vegetables and a little salt and pepper. Stir the tomato purée into the stock. Pour over the meat and vegetables.
4. Return the casserole to the oven, reduce the temperature to 350°F and cook for about 1,5 hours until the meat is tender.
5. To make the dumplings, mix together the flour, suet and seasoning with enough water to form a stiff dough. This makes about 6 small dumplings.
6. Add the dumplings to the hotpot for the last 30 minutes of cooking.

Green Chilli & Meat Stew

Ingredients:

- 212lb stewing beef, cubed
- 1.2 litres/2pt water
- 100g/4oz fresh green chillies, roasted, peeled, seeded and chopped
- 2 teaspoons garlic powder
- 1 teaspoon cornflour
- salt
- freshly ground black pepper

Procedure:

1. Cover the meat with water in a large heavy pan, bring to the boil and simmer gently for 4 hours.
2. Add the chillies and garlic powder Season with salt and pepper.

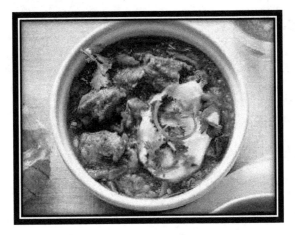

3. Dissolve the cornflour in
4. 2 teaspoons water to form a paste, and stir in rapidly. When the mixture has thickened, simmer for about 45 minutes. Serve hot.

Beef & Stout Casserole

Serves 4

Ingredients:

- 1,5 lb beef
- 6 oz lean bacon, cubed
- 1 tablespoon vegetable oil
- 1/2 oz butter
- 2 tablespoons plain flour
- 1 bottle of stout
- 1 lb shallots
- 3 garlic cloves, crushed
- 1 tablespoon sugar
- 1 tablespoon wine or cider vinegar
- salt
- freshly ground black pepper

Procedure:

1. Preheat the oven to 300°F.

2. Sauté the beef and bacon in the oil. Drain off the excess liquid. Remove the meat and set aside.

3. Add the butter to the pan and melt. Stir in the flour to make a roux; cook, stirring, for a minute or two.

4. Gradually stir in the stout.

5. Put the meat and the shallots in a deep casserole dish, and season with salt and pepper.

6. Add the garlic. Sprinkle the sugar on top, and pour in the sauce.

7. Cover and put in the oven. Cook very gently for up to 3 hours.

8. Remove from the oven and mix in the vinegar. Serve hot with boiled potatoes.

Rabbit Hotpot

Serves 4

Ingredients:

- 2 lb rabbit, jointed
- 2 onions, sliced
- 2 tablespoons wholegrain mustard
- 12 prunes, pitted
- 4 bay leaves
- ¾pt dry cider
- ¾ pt chicken stock
- 4 tablespoons plain flour, seasoned with salt and freshly ground black pepper
- 2 tablespoons vegetable oil
- 1/2 oz butter
- 1 lb parsnips, cut into chunks
- 14 oz canned cooked kidney beans, drained

Procedure:

1. Put the rabbit joints, onions, mustard, prunes and bay leaves into a bowl, cover with the cider and stock.
2. Mix, cover tightly, and marinate in the refrigerator overnight.
3. Preheat the oven to 350°F.
4. Remove the rabbit joints and prunes from the marinade; reserve.
5. Pat the rabbit dry with kitchen paper, and dredge in the seasoned flour.
6. Heat the oil and butter in a large flameproof casserole dish, add the joints and fry until browned. Sprinkle with any remaining flour.
7. Add the reserved marinade and the parsnips, and bring to the boil.
8. Cover and transfer to the oven. Bake for 40 minutes.
9. Add the prunes and kidney beans, and bake for 20–30 minutes until tender.
10. Serve hot.

Mexican Nacho Casserole

Ingredients:

- 1 lb minced beef
- 1 tablespoon dried mixed herbs
- 4 oz canned refried beans
- 2 oz onions, chopped
- 7 oz nacho chips
- 1 green pepper, seeded and diced
- 4 oz Cheddar cheese, grated

Procedure:

1. Preheat the oven to 400°F.
2. Cook the minced beef and herbs in a frying pan, mixing well and stirring to break up any lumps.

3. Spread the refried beans in the bottom of a medium casserole dish, then sprinkle with the onions.

4. Layer the meat over the beans. Bake in the oven for 15 minutes.

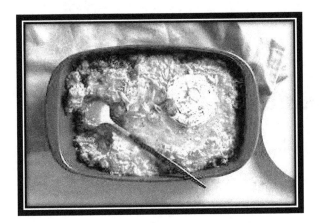

5. Tuck the nacho chips around the edges of the casserole, then top with the pepper and cheese, and bake for a further 5 minutes.

6. Serve immediately.

One-Pot Beef Dinner

Serves 6

Ingredients:

- 3 tablespoons vegetable oil
- 1 small onion, chopped
- 1 large egg, lightly beaten
- 450g/1lb minced beef
- 50g/2oz plain breadcrumbs
- 112 teaspoons onion powder
- 112 teaspoons garlic salt
- 4 medium potatoes, sliced
- 450g/1lb frozen carrots

Procedure:

1. Heat the oil in a frying pan over a medium-high heat. Reduce the heat to medium once the oil is hot. Add the onion to the pan, and sweat until soft.

2. In a large bowl, mix the egg, beef, 50ml/2fl oz water, breadcrumbs, onion powder and garlic salt. Press the meat into the bottom of the bowl to form a rounded loaf. Invert the bowl to remove, and put the loaf on top of the onion. Put the sliced potatoes around the loaf and the carrots on top of the potatoes.

3. Sprinkle with additional seasonings if desired. Cover and cook for about 1 hour. After 30 minutes, turn the meatloaf over and stir the vegetables. Serve hot.

Lamb Hotpot

Ingredients:

- 1,5 lb lean lamb neck cutlets
- 5 fl oz lamb stock
- 2 lamb's kidneys
- 1 oz butter, melted
- 1,5 lb potatoes, thinly sliced
- salt
- freshly ground black
- 1 large onion, thinly sliced pepper
- 2 tablespoons chopped fresh thyme

Procedure:

1. Preheat the oven to 350°F.
2. Remove any excess fat from the lamb. Skin and core the kidneys, and cut them into slices.
3. Arrange a layer of potatoes in the bottom of a 3 pt ovenproof dish.
4. Arrange the lamb neck cutlets on top of the potatoes, and cover with the kidneys, onion and thyme.
5. Pour the stock over the meat, and season with salt and pepper.
6. Layer the remaining potato slices on top, overlapping to completely cover the meat and onion.
7. Brush the potato slices with the butter, cover the dish and cook in the oven for 1,5 hours.
8. Remove the lid and cook for a further 30 minutes until golden brown on top.
9. Serve hot.

Ulster Irish Stew

<u>Serves 4</u>

Ingredients:

- 900g/2lb neck of lamb, cubed
- 900g/2lb potatoes, sliced
- 450g/1lb onions, thickly sliced
- 1 sprig of fresh thyme
- salt
- freshly ground black pepper

Procedure:

1. Layer the meat, potatoes and onion in a casserole dish, seasoning each layer well with salt and pepper.
2. Finish with a layer of potatoes.

3. Fill to about two-thirds full with water, add the thyme and cover with a lid.

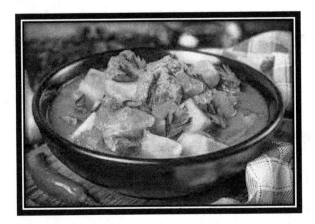

4. Bring to the boil and simmer for 1–2 hours until the lamb is really tender.
5. Serve hot.

Lamb & Vegetable Stew

<u>Serves 4</u>

Ingredients:

- 2 tablespoons olive oil
- 400g/14oz lean lamb fillet, cubed
- 1 red onion, sliced
- 1 garlic clove, crushed
- 1 potato, cubed
- 400g/14oz canned chopped plum tomatoes
- 1 red pepper, seeded and chopped
- 200g/7oz canned chickpeas
- 1 aubergine, cut into chunks
- 200ml/7fl oz lamb stock
- 1 tablespoon red wine vinegar
- 1 teaspoon chopped fresh thyme
- 1 teaspoon chopped fresh rosemary
- 1 teaspoon chopped fresh oregano

- 8 pitted black olives, halved
- salt
- ground black pepper

Procedure:

1. Preheat the oven to 325°F.
2. Heat 1 tablespoon of the oil in a flameproof casserole dish and, over a high heat, brown the lamb.
3. Reduce the heat and add the remaining oil, the onion and the garlic. Cook until soft.
4. Add the potato, tomatoes, pepper, drained chickpeas, aubergine, stock, vinegar and herbs to the casserole dish.
5. Season with salt and pepper, stir and bring to the boil.
6. Cover and cook in the oven for 1–1½ hours until tender.
7. About 15 minutes before the end of cooking time, add the olives.
8. Serve hot.

Irish Hotpot

<u>Serves 6</u>

Ingredients:

- 6 potatoes, thinly sliced
- 2 onions, thinly sliced
- 3 carrots, thinly sliced
- 3 oz cooked long-grain rice
- 14 oz canned peas
- 1 lb 5oz pork and herb sausages
- 15 oz canned condensed tomato soup, diluted
- salt
- freshly ground black pepper

Procedure:

1. Preheat the oven to 375°F.
2. Layer the potatoes, onions and carrots in a large casserole dish, seasoning as you go with salt and pepper.
3. Sprinkle with the rice and peas, and top with the sausages. Pour the diluted soup over all.
4. Bake in the oven, covered, for 1 hour.
5. Remove the lid from the casserole, turn the sausages and bake, uncovered, for a further 1 hour.
6. Serve hot.

Sausage & Sweet Pepper Casserole

Serves 4–6

Ingredients:

- 2 tablespoons olive oil
- 1 lb spicy sausages, cut into 5cm/2in slices
- 1,5 lb green peppers, seeded and sliced
- 8 oz tomatoes, skinned and quartered
- 1 teaspoon chopped fresh flat-leaf parsley
- salt
- freshly ground black pepper

Procedure:

1. Heat the oil in a pan, and gently fry the sausages until lightly browned.

2. Add the peppers, and fry for a further 3 minutes, stirring continuously.

3. Add the tomatoes and parsley to the pan. Season with salt and pepper.

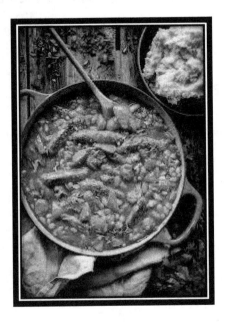

4. Cover the pan and cook gently for about 10 minutes until the sausages are cooked through.

5. Serve hot.

Tuscan Veal Broth

Ingredients:

- 2 oz dried peas, soaked for
- 2 hours and drained
- 2 lb boned neck of veal, diced
- 2 pt beef stock
- 2 oz barley
- 1 carrot, diced
- 1 turnip, diced
- 1 leek, thinly sliced
- 1 red onion, finely chopped
- 4 oz tomatoes, chopped
- 1 sprig of fresh basil
- 4 oz dried vermicelli
- salt
- freshly ground black pepper

Procedure:

1. Put the peas, veal, stock and 600ml/1pt water in a large pan. Bring to the boil over a low heat.

2. Using a slotted spoon, skim off any scum that rises to the surface.

3. When all the scum has been removed, add the barley and a pinch of salt. Simmer gently over a low heat for 25 minutes.

4. Add the carrot, turnip, leek, onion, tomatoes and basil to the pan, and season with salt and pepper.

5. Leave to simmer for about 2 hours, skimming the surface from time to time to remove any scum.

6. Remove the pan from the heat and set aside for 2 hours.

7. Set the pan over a medium heat and bring to the boil. Add the vermicelli and cook for 12 minutes.

8. Season with salt and pepper, then remove and discard the basil.

9. Serve immediately.

Bacon & Lentil Stew

Ingredients:

- 1 lb rindless smoked back bacon rashers, diced
- 1 onion, chopped
- 2 carrots, sliced
- 2 celery sticks, chopped
- 1 turnip, chopped
- 1 large potato, chopped
- 3 oz green lentils such as Puy, rinsed and drained
- 1 bouquet garni
- 1,5 pt chicken stock
- salt
- freshly ground black pepper

Procedure:

1. Heat a large flameproof casserole and add the bacon.
2. Cook over a medium heat, stirring, for 5 minutes or until the fat runs.
3. Add the onion, carrots, celery, turnip and potato, and cook, stirring, for 5 minutes.
4. Add the lentils, bouquet garni and stock.
5. Bring to the boil, reduce the heat andsimmer for 1 hour or until the lentils are tender.
6. Remove and discard the bouquet garni, and season with salt and pepper.
7. Serve immediately.

One-Pot Pork Chop Supper

Ingredients:

- 1 tablespoon vegetable oil
- 4 pork chops
- 14 oz canned tomato soup
- 1 teaspoon Worcestershire sauce
- 1/2 teaspoon salt
- 1/2 teaspoon caraway seeds
- 3 potatoes, quartered
- 4 carrots, cut into 2 in pieces

Procedure:

1. In a large frying pan, brown the chops in the oil.

2. Pour off any fat, then add the soup, 4 fl oz water, Worcestershire sauce, salt, caraway, potatoes and carrots.

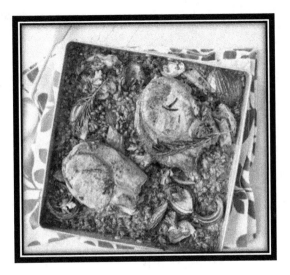

3. Cover and simmer for 45 minutes or until tender.

4. Serve hot.

Ham & Cheese Casserole

Serves 8

Ingredients:

- 4 oz plain flour
- 3 oz butter
- 1 pt milk
- 11 oz ham, chopped
- 1 lb 5oz potatoes, thinly sliced
- 9 oz Cheddar cheese, grated
- 1 onion, chopped
- 1 green pepper, seeded and chopped
- salt
- freshly ground black pepper

Procedure:

1. Preheat the oven to 350°F.
2. Season the flour with salt and pepper. Melt the butter in a saucepan, then add the flour mixture.
3. Cook over a medium heat for 1 minute, stirring constantly.
4. Remove from the heat and stir in the milk. Return to the heat and cook until thick.
5. In a very large bowl, mix the remaining ingredients with the sauce.
6. Bake in a casserole dish for 1,5 hours, keeping the casserole covered for the first 30 minutes of cooking.
7. Allow to cool for 15 minutes before serving.

Pot Roast Of Venison

Serves 4

Ingredients:

- 4 lb boned joint of venison
- 3 fl oz vegetable oil
- 4 cloves
- 8 black peppercorns, lightly crushed
- 9 fl oz red wine
- 4 oz streaky back bacon, chopped
- 2 onions, finely chopped
- 2 carrots, chopped
- 5 oz mushrooms, sliced
- 1 tablespoon plain flour
- 9 fl oz chicken stock
- 2 tablespoons redcurrant jelly
- salt
- freshly ground black pepper

Procedure:

1. Put the venison in a bowl, add half of the oil, the spices and wine, cover and leave in a cool place for 24 hours, turning the meat occasionally.

2. Preheat the oven to 325°F.

3. Remove the venison from the bowl and pat dry with kitchen paper.

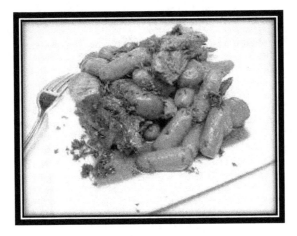

4. Reserve the marinade. Heat the remaining oil in a shallow pan, then brown the venison evenly. Transfer to a plate.

5. Stir the bacon, onions, carrot and mushrooms into the pan, and cook for about 5 minutes.

6. Stir in the flour and cook for 2 minutes, then remove from the heat and stir in the marinade, stock and redcurrant jelly. Season with salt and pepper.

7. Return to the heat and bring to the boil, stirring, then simmer for 2–3 minutes.

8. Transfer the venison and sauce to a casserole dish, cover and cook in the oven, turning the joint occasionally, for about 3 hours until tender.

9. Serve hot.

Veal & Spinach Stew

Ingredients:

- 2 lb loin of veal, chopped into 1 in cubes
- 2 lb spinach
- 2 onions, chopped
- 1 oz butter
- salt
- freshly ground black pepper

Procedure:

1. Put all the ingredients in a large casserole dish.
2. Pour in 8fl oz water, cover and cook over a high heat for about 35 minutes.
3. Serve hot.

Pheasant & Wild Rice Casserole

Serves 6

Ingredients:

- 14 oz pheasant, diced
- 9 oz wild rice
- 8 oz mushrooms, sliced
- 3 oz butter
- 1 onion, chopped
- 2 oz plain flour
- 10 fl oz chicken stock
- 10 fl oz milk
- 2 tablespoons chopped fresh flat-leaf parsley
- 2 oz slivered almonds, toasted
- salt
- freshly ground black pepper

Procedure:

1. Preheat the oven to 350°F

2. Poach the pheasant in simmering water for 1 hour or until tender.

3. Prepare the rice according to the packet instructions.

4. Sauté the mushrooms in half of the butter, then remove from the pan and reserve.

5. Sauté the onion in the remaining butter until softened.

6. Remove from the heat, and stir in the flour until smooth.

7. Gradually stir the stock into the flour mixture, then add the milk.

8. Return to the heat and cook, stirring constantly, until thick.

9. Add the rice, mushrooms, pheasant and parsley, and season with salt and pepper.

10. Transfer the mixture to a large casserole dish, and sprinkle with the almonds.

11. Bake in the oven for 25–30 minutes.

12. Serve hot.

Baked bean & bacon casserole

<u>Serves 3</u>

Ingredients:

- 6 rashers rindless back bacon
- 1 lb canned baked beans
- 2 tablespoons minced onion
- 2 tablespoons tomato ketchup
- 1 teaspoon prepared mustard
- 2 tablespoons Demerara sugar

Procedure:

1. Preheat the oven to 375°F.
2. Dry-fry the bacon in a frying pan until very crisp.

3. In a deep casserole dish, combine the beans, onion, ketchup, mustard and sugar. Mix thoroughly.

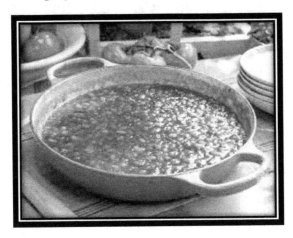

4. Crumble the bacon, and sprinkle over the baked bean mixture.
5. Heat in the oven, uncovered, for 10 minutes or until the sauce is bubbly.
6. Serve hot.

Liver & Macaroni Casserole

Serves 4

Ingredients:

- 12 oz pigs' livers, thinly sliced
- 1 oz butter
- 2 onions, thinly sliced
- 3 tablespoons plain flour
- 5 fl oz chicken stock
- 14 oz canned chopped plum tomatoes
- 2 teaspoons chopped fresh sage
- 4 oz macaroni
- salt
- freshly ground black pepper

Procedure:

1. Preheat the oven to 350°F.

2. Brown the liver in half the butter in a flameproof casserole dish for 1 minute on each side.

3. Remove from the pan with a slotted spoon.

4. Add the remaining butter, and sauté the onions for 3 minutes until soft and lightly golden

5. Add the flour and cook, stirring, for 1 minute.

6. Blend in the stock and tomatoes. Bring to the boil, stirring, for 1 minute.

7. Return the liver to the pan and add the sage and a little salt and pepper.

8. Cover and cook in the oven for 1 hour.

9. Cook the pasta until al dente. Drain. Stir into the casserole.

10. Serve hot.

Rabbit Casserole

Serves 4

Ingredients:

- 25g/1oz butter
- 900g/2lb rabbit pieces
- 200g/7oz tomatoes
- 1 tablespoon cornflour
- 100g/4oz carrot, coarsely grated
- 1 teaspoon dried oregano
- 50ml/2fl oz brandy
- 25ml/1fl oz white wine vinegar
- 375ml/13fl oz warm water 2 bay leaves
- 1 tablespoon finely grated orange zest

Procedure:

1. Preheat the oven to 350°F.

2. Melt the butter in a large frying pan and brown the rabbit pieces well, turning frequently, then transfer the pieces to a large casserole dish.

3. Put the tomatoes in a bowl of boiling water; leave for 2 minutes.

4. Peel off the skins and chop the flesh into small cubes. Add to the casserole dish.

5. Combine the cornflour, carrot, orange zest and oregano in a small bowl. Pour in the brandy, vinegar and warm water, and stir well.

6. Pour over the contents of the casserole dish and add the bay leaves.

7. Cover and bake for 112 hours or until the rabbit is tender.

8. Serve hot.

Swiss chicken casserole

Ingredients:

- 500g/1lb 5oz cooked chicken, chopped into bite-size pieces
- 175g/6oz celery, sliced
- 200g/7oz herb stuffing, broken up
- 225ml/8fl oz salad dressing
- 125ml/4fl oz milk
- 50g/2oz onion, chopped
- 225g/8oz Emmenthaler cheese, grated
- 50g/2oz toasted slivered almonds
- salt and freshly ground black pepper

Procedure:

1. Preheat the oven to 350°F.
2. Combine the chicken, celery, stuffing, salad dressing, milk, onion and cheese in a large casserole dish.
3. Season with salt and pepper, and sprinkle with the almonds.

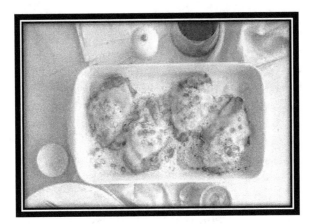

4. Cover the casserole with a lid and bake in the oven for 25 minutes.
5. Remove the lid and continue baking for a further 10 minutes.
6. Serve hot.

Chicken & Potato Bake

<u>Serves 4</u>

Ingredients:

- 2 tablespoons olive oil
- 4 chicken breasts
- 1 bunch of spring onions, trimmed and chopped
- 12 oz carrots, sliced
- 4 oz green beans, trimmed and sliced
- 1 pt chicken stock
- 12 oz new potatoes
- 2 tablespoons cornflour
- salt
- freshly ground black pepper

Procedure:

1. Preheat the oven to 375°F.

2. Heat the oil in a large flameproof casserole dish, and add the chicken breasts.

3. Gently fry for 5–8 minutes until browned on both sides. Lift from the casserole dish with a slotted spoon and set aside.

4. Add the spring onions, carrots and green beans to the dish, and gently fry for 3–4 minutes.

5. Return the chicken to the casserole dish, and pour in the stock.

6. Add the potatoes, season with salt and pepper, and bring to the boil.

7. Cover the casserole dish, transfer to the oven and bake for 40–50 minutes until the potatoes are tender.

8. Blend the cornflour with 3 tablespoons cold water. Add to the casserole, stirring until blended and thickened.

9. Cover and cook for a further 5 minutes. Serve immediately.

Liver Hotpot

<u>Serves 6</u>

Ingredients:

- 1 lb 2oz lamb's liver
- 1 oz plain flour
- 2 large onions, thinly sliced
- 1,75 lb potatoes,
- thinly sliced
- 18 fl oz lamb stock
- 6 rashers streaky bacon
- salt
- freshly ground black pepper

Procedure:

1. Preheat the oven to 350°F. Lightly grease a large casserole dish.Remove the skin and tubes from the liver.

2. Season the flour with salt and pepper. Dredge each slice of liver in the seasoned flour.

3. Arrange layers of liver, onion and potatoes in the casserole dish, ending with a neat layer of potatoes.

4. Heat the stock and pour in just enough to cover the potatoes.

5. Cover the casserole dish and bake for about 1 hour until the liver is tender.

6. Remove the lid and arrange the bacon rashers on top. Continue cooking, uncovered, until the bacon is crisp.

7. Serve hot.

Woodpigeon Casserole

<u>Serves 4</u>

Ingredients:

- 2 pig's trotters
- 1 oz butter
- 1 tablespoon vegetable oil
- 4 woodpigeon
- 12 pickling onions
- 1 carrot, diced
- 1 celery stick, diced
- 4 oz streaky back bacon, cut into strips
- 1 cinnamon stick
- 1 bay leaf
- 2 sprigs of fresh thyme
- 1,5 tablespoons plain flour

- 16 prunes, pitted
- 2 sprigs of fresh flat-leaf parsley
- 10 fl oz red wine
- salt
- freshly ground black pepper

Procedure:

1. Put the trotters in a pan and cover with water. Bring to the boil, cover and simmer for 1 hour, skimming off any scum that rises to the surface.
2. Reserve the liquid and trotters.
3. Melt the butter and oil in a flameproof casserole dish. Quickly brown the pigeons, then remove and reserve.
4. Add the onions, carrot, celery and bacon to the pan with the cinnamon, bay leaf and thyme.
5. Stir to coat with the fat, then reduce the heat, cover and sweat gently for 10 minutes.
6. Sprinkle with the flour and stir.

7. Return the pigeons to the pan, together with the trotters, prunes, parsley, wine and 1 pt of the reserved cooking liquid.

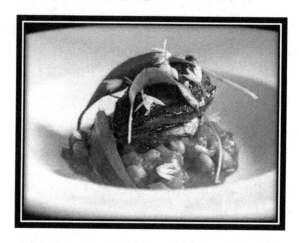

8. Season lightly with salt and pepper.
9. Bring to the boil, cover and simmer gently, turning the pigeons occasionally, for 45–60 minutes, until tender.
10. Serve hot.

Hare Stew

Serves 6

Ingredients:

- 8 oz smoked back bacon, cut into strips
- 4 fl oz olive oil
- 8 oz onions, sliced
- 2 garlic cloves, chopped
- plain flour for dredging
- 4 lb hare, cut into 12 pieces
- 1 pt red wine
- 1 pt chicken stock
- 1 bouquet garni
- 24 pickling onions
- 1 oz butter
- 8 oz button mushrooms

- 2 tablespoons chopped fresh flat-leaf parsley
- salt
- freshly ground black pepper

Procedure:

1. Fry the bacon slowly in 2 tablespoons of the oil until almost crisp, then transfer to a casserole dish with a slotted spoon.
2. Fry the onions in this fat until soft and translucent.
3. Add the garlic and cook for a further 2 minutes, then add the onions and garlic to the casserole dish.
4. Season the hare with salt and pepper, and dredge in the flour.
5. Add 2 tablespoons of the oil to the pan, increase the heat to medium and brown the hare pieces on all sides. Transfer to the casserole dish.

6. Increase the heat under the frying pan, add the wine and deglaze, scraping up any bits clinging to the pan.

7. Pour the wine mixture over the hare ,and add the stock, bouquet garni and salt and pepper.

8. Bring to the boil, skim off any scum that rises to the surface, then reduce the heat, cover and simmer for about 1 hour.

9. About 15 minutes before the end of the cooking time, fry the pickling onions in the butter and remaining oil.

10. Season lightly with salt and pepper, and sauté for 5–10 minutes until golden brown.

11. Transfer to a dish and keep warm while you fry the button mushrooms.

12. Add these to the onions, and stir both into the casserole dish.

13. Scatter the parsley over the top, and serve hot.

One-Pot Chicken Couscous

Serves 8

Ingredients:

- 2 lb boneless, skinless chicken breasts, cut into 1 in chunks
- 2 fl oz olive oil
- 4 large carrots, peeled and sliced
- 2 onions, diced
- 3 garlic cloves, crushed
- 1 lb 2oz canned chicken soup
- 9 oz couscous
- 2 teaspoons Tabasco sauce
- 1/2 teaspoon salt
- 7 oz raisins
- 7 oz slivered almonds, toasted
- 2 oz fresh parsley, chopped

70

Procedure:

1. In a large frying pan over a medium-high heat, cook the chicken in the oil until well browned on all sides.
2. Using a slotted spoon, remove the chicken to a plate.
3. Reduce the heat to medium.
4. In the remaining drippings, cook the carrots and onion for 5 minutes.
5. Add the garlic and cook for a further 2 minutes, stirring frequently.
6. Add the soup, Tabasco sauce, salt and chicken. Bring to the boil, then reduce the heat to low, cover and simmer for 5 minutes.
7. Stir in the raisins, almonds and parsley.
8. Heat through, and serve immediately.

Venison & Wild Rice Casserole

Ingredients:

- 13 fl oz cream of mushroom soup
- 3 oz button mushrooms
- 9 oz wild rice
- 6 lean venison chops
- 1 medium onion, thinly sliced
- 3 rashers lean back bacon
- salt
- freshly ground black pepper

Procedure:

1. Preheat the oven to 350°F.
2. Put 18 fl oz water, the soup and the mushrooms in a large casserole dish.

3. Rinse the rice in cold water a few times, drain and add to the casserole dish. Spread the venison chops out in the sauce.

4. Season with salt and pepper, and arrange the onions on top, then the bacon.

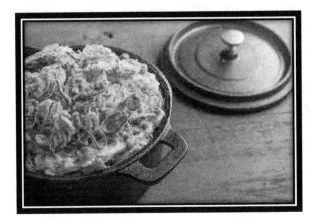

5. Cover and bake in the oven for 1–1,5 hours until the meat and rice are soft and cooked.

6. Serve hot.

Spanish partridge & chocolate stew

<u>Serves 4</u>

Ingredients:

- 2 partridges, halved
- 2 tablespoons olive oil
- 1 large onion, chopped
- 8 garlic cloves
- 2 cloves
- 1 bay leaf
- 10 fl oz dry white wine
- 1 tablespoon sherry vinegar
- 1 oz plain chocolate, grated
- salt
- freshly ground black pepper

Procedure:

1. Brown the partridges in the oil in a frying pan over a high heat, and transfer to a casserole dish.

2. Fry the onion in the same oil, then transfer to the casserole dish.

3. Add all the remaining ingredients to the casserole dish except the chocolate, and bring to a gentle simmer, cover tightly and continue simmering for 45–50 minutes until the partridges are tender.

4. Transfer the meat to a serving dish and keep warm.

5. Stir the chocolate into the remaining liquid in the pan, and simmer for a further 3 minutes. Stir and adjust the seasoning.

6. Pour the sauce over the partridges, and serve immediately.

Pumpkin Turkey Stew

<u>Serves 6</u>

Ingredients:

- 2 tablespoons canola oil
- 4 onions, finely chopped
- 2 teaspoons grated fresh root ginger
- 1,5 lb skinless turkey thigh fillet, cut into 1,5 in cubes
- 14 oz canned chopped plum tomatoes
- 7 oz pumpkin purée
- 1/2 teaspoon salt
- 1/4 teaspoon pepper
- 2 tablespoons chopped fresh coriander leaves

Procedure:

1. Heat 1 tablespoon of the oil in a large flameproof casserole dish over a medium heat.

2. Sweat the onions for 3 minutes until softened.

3. Add the ginger and cook for a further 2 minutes. Transfer to a bowl.

4. Heat the remaining oil in the casserole dish.

5. Brown the turkey in batches, allowing 3–4 minutes per batch. Return the onions and ginger to the casserole dish.

6. Stir in the tomatoes, pumpkin purée, salt, pepper and 8 fl oz water. Bring to the boil.

7. Reduce the heat to low and simmer, part-covered, for 40 minutes, until the turkey is tender. Stir occasionally.

8. Add the coriander and cook for a further 2 minutes, then serve hot.

Grouse Stew

Ingredients:

- 1 grouse, cut into bite-size pieces plain flour for dredging
- 1 oz butter
- 3 pt boiling water 1 teaspoon dried thyme
- 7 oz sweetcorn
- 2 potatoes, cubed
- 1/4 teaspoon cayenne pepper
- 3 onions, sliced
- 14 oz canned chopped plum tomatoes
- salt
- freshly ground black pepper

Procedure:

1. Roll the grouse pieces in the flour seasoned with salt and pepper.
2. Melt the butter in a large heavy frying pan, and brown the grouse on all sides.
3. Put the grouse and all the other ingredients except the tomatoes in a large casserole dish.
4. Add the boiling water, then cover and simmer for 1,5–2 hours.
5. Add the tomatoes and continue to simmer for a further 1 hour.
6. Serve hot.

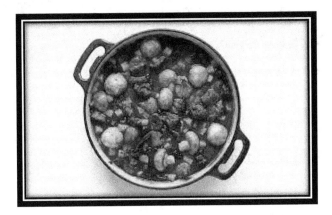

Quail Stew

Ingredients:

- 8 medium quails
- 1 tablespoon ground cumin 1 tablespoon vegetable oil 15g/12oz butter
- 2 large onions, finely chopped
- 1 tablespoon crushed garlic
- 1 teaspoon tomato purée 1 teaspoon allspice
- 4 green cardamom pods
- salt
- ground black pepper

Procedure:

1. Wash the quails thoroughly inside and out, removing all fat from the tops and bottoms of the quails.
2. Cut each quail in two, with bottoms and chests separated. Season with the cumin.
3. In a large cooking pan, heat the oil and butter.
4. Add the onions and garlic, and stir until the onions begin to brown.
5. Put the quails in the pan, turning to brown all over.
6. Next, add the tomato purée, cover the pan and reduce the heat. Season with salt and pepper, and add the allspice, cardamom and enough boiling water just to keep a thick sauce.
7. Leave to cook for 30 minutes until well done.
8. Remove the cardamom, and serve hot.

Oyster & Cauliflower Stew

Ingredients:

- 1 oz butter
- 1 pt canned shucked oysters with liquid
- 4 oz cauliflower florets, blanched
- 1 tablespoon cornflour
- 14 fl oz milk
- 1/4 teaspoon salt
- 1/4 teaspoon cracked black pepper
- 1/4 teaspoon onion powder

Procedure:

1. Put the butter in a large microwave-safe baking dish. Cover with kitchen paper.
2. Heat in the microwave on high for 45 seconds or until melted.
3. Drain the oysters, reserving the liquid. Add the oysters to the butter, and cook on high for 1 minute.
4. Using a slotted spoon, remove the oysters to a container or pot with the cauliflower.
5. Gradually add the cornflour to the oyster liquid, and stir until blended.
6. Add the milk and transfer the liquid to the baking dish.
7. Add the salt, pepper and onion powder.
8. Cook on high for 4–5 minutes until slightly thickened, stirring twice.
9. Add the oysters and cauliflower to the dish, and cook on high for 2 minutes.
10. Serve hot.

Pheasant Casserole

Ingredients:

- 2 tablespoons beef dripping
- 2 pheasants, jointed, breast and legs only
- 1 onion, chopped
- 1 carrot, chopped
- 1 celery stick, chopped
- 12 fl oz red wine
- salt
- freshly ground black pepper

Procedure:

1. Preheat the oven to 350°F.
2. Heat the dripping in a frying pan and brown the pheasant joints.

3. Remove from the pan, and put in a casserole dish.

4. Put the vegetables in the frying pan, and cook for 2 minutes, then add the red wine and bring to the boil.

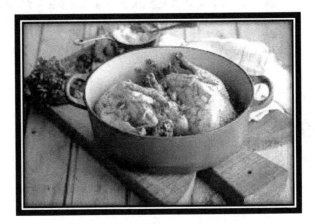

5. Pour the mixture over the pheasant joints, season with salt and pepper, and cover the casserole dish.

6. Cook in the oven for 1–1,5 hours until tender.

7. Serve hot.

Aubergine, Mozzarella & Cheddar Hotpot

Ingredients:

- 4 large white potatoes, thinly sliced
- 2 tablespoons olive oil
- 1 aubergine, sliced
- 1 large onion, sliced
- 10 oz canned chopped plum tomatoes
- 15 oz canned cooked chickpeas, drained
- 1 oz green lentils such as Puy, picked and rinsed
- 2 garlic cloves, crushed
- 2 tablespoons chopped fresh flat-leaf parsley
- 1 oz mozzarella cheese, finely grated
- 1 oz Cheddar cheese, finely grated

- 1 tablespoon boiling water
- salt
- freshly ground black pepper

Procedure:

1. Put the potatoes in a saucepan of salted cold water.
2. Bring to the boil, and cook until beginning to soften – do not cook completely. Drain and set aside.
3. Heat the oil in a frying pan and gently sauté the aubergine until it begins to brown. Turn and repeat on the other side.
4. As each piece is done, remove to kitchen paper.
5. When the aubergine is cooked, stir the onion in the frying pan until softened, but not browned.
6. Stir in the tomatoes, chickpeas, lentils, garlic, parsley and seasoning.

7. Cook over a medium heat for 40 to 45 minutes, or until the lentils are tender.

8. Preheat the oven to 400°F.

9. Mix the cheeses together. Add the boiling water to make a paste.

10. When the tomato mixture is ready, spoon the remaining mixture over the bottom of a large casserole dish.

11. Cover with half the aubergine and add another third of the tomato mixture. Layer on the remaining aubergine.

12. Spread a third of the cheese mixture on to the aubergine.

13. Add half the potatoes, another third of the cheese and then the remaining potatoes.

14. Finish with the final third of cheese.

15. Cover and bake in the middle of oven for 30 minutes.

16. Remove the lid and bake for a further 10 minutes to brown.

Duck & Pomegranate Stew

Ingredients:

- 2 small pomegranates
- 4 lb duck, cut into 8 pieces
- 3 tablespoons sunflower oil
- 1 onion, chopped
- 8 oz shelled walnuts, coarsely ground
- 3/4 pt chicken stock
- 1 cinnamon stick
- 2 cloves
- juice of 1/2 lemon
- pinch of granulated sugar
- salt
- freshly ground black pepper

Procedure.

1. Squeeze the juice from one of the pomegranates using a lemon squeezer. Extract the seeds of the other pomegranate and reserve.

2. Brown the duck pieces briskly in half of the oil, and transfer to a flameproof casserole dish. Fry the onion in the same fat until it is tender, and transfer to the casserole dish.

3. Add the walnuts to the pan, and fry until they begin to change colour, then scrape into the casserole dish.

4. Return the frying pan to the heat and pour in the stock. Bring to the boil, stirring up any pan residue.

5. Pour into the casserole dish and add the cinnamon stick, cloves, pomegranate juice, lemon juice and sugar. Season with salt and pepper.

6. Cover and simmer for 30 minutes.

7. Remove the lid and continue simmering, uncovered, for 20–30 minutes until the meat is very tender and the sauce is thick.

8. Taste and adjust the seasoning, and serve hot with the pomegranate seeds sprinkled over the top.

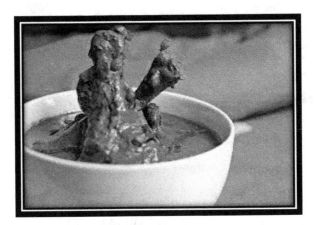

Chinese Vegetable Casserole

Ingredients:

- 4 tablespoons vegetable oil
- 2 carrots, sliced
- 1 courgette, sliced
- 4 baby sweetcorn, halved lengthways
- 4 oz cauliflower florets
- 1 leek, sliced
- 4 oz water chestnuts, halved
- 8 oz firm tofu, diced
- 10 fl oz vegetable stock 1 teaspoon salt
- 2 teaspoons soft dark brown sugar such as muscovado
- 2 teaspoons light soy sauce
- 2 tablespoons dry sherry

- 1 tablespoon cornflour
- 1 tablespoon chopped fresh coriander leaves, to garnish

Procedure:

1. Heat the oil in a preheated wok until it is almost smoking.
2. Reduce the heat slightly, and add the carrots, courgette, sweetcorn, cauliflower and leek. Stir-fry for 2–3 minutes.
3. Stir in the water chestnuts, tofu, stock, salt, sugar, soy sauce and sherry, and bring to the boil.
4. Reduce the heat, cover and simmer for 20 minutes.
5. Blend the cornflour with 2 tablespoons water to form a smooth paste.
6. Stir the paste into the wok, bring the sauce to the boil and cook, stirring constantly, until it thickens and turns glossy.
7. To serve, scatter the coriander over the top, and serve immediately.

Guinea Fowl Stew

Ingredients:

- 2 fl oz groundnut oil
- 2 lb guinea fowl, cut into bite-size pieces
- 1 teaspoon dried thyme
- 1 teaspoon curry powder
- 2 large onions, sliced
- 8 oz fresh red chillies, seeded and chopped
- 2 lb tomatoes
- 8 oz tomato purée
- 2 garlic cloves
- 2 onions, sliced

Procedure:

1. In a large frying pan, heat half of the oil and brown the guinea fowl pieces, in batches if necessary, with the thyme and curry powder.
2. Remove to a plate and keep warm.
3. Add the remaining oil to the pan and sweat the onions and chillies for a few minutes, then add the tomatoes and cook for about 20 minutes until fairly dry.
4. Add the tomato purée, stir thoroughly and add the guinea fowl pieces.
5. Simmer gently for another 10 minutes, stirring frequently.
6. Serve hot.

Trout Stew

Serves 4

Ingredients:

- 1 teaspoon salt
- 1 onion, thinly sliced
- 8 fl oz tomato juice
- 2 garlic cloves, crushed
- 4 small potatoes, diced
- 1 green pepper, seeded and chopped
- 1 medium tomato, peeled and chopped
- 2,5 lb trout fillets
- 10 oz frozen green beans

Procedure:

1. Combine all the ingredients except the trout and green beans in a large microwave-safe casserole dish.

2. Add 2 fl oz water. Cover and microwave for 10 minutes on high or until the potatoes are tender.

3. Add the fish and green beans to the stew, cover, and microwave for a further 5 minutes on high.

4. Let stand for a minute or two before serving.

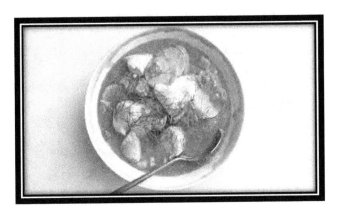

Turkey, Pea & Ham Pot Pie

Serves 6

Ingredients:

- 2 oz plain flour
- 1 lb 2oz turkey thighs, diced
- 4 tablespoons vegetable oil
- 1 onion, chopped
- 9 fl oz chicken stock
- 175g/6oz ham, cut into
- bite-size chunks
- 5 oz frozen peas
- 2 teaspoons chopped fresh tarragon
- 2 teaspoons chopped fresh chives
- 2 tablespoons crème fraîche
- 13 oz ready-rolled puff pastry

- 1 egg, beaten
- salt
- freshly ground black pepper

Procedure:

1. Preheat the oven to 400°F.

2. Put the flour in a bowl, season with salt and pepper, and toss the turkey until coated.

3. Heat half of the oil in a large frying pan and brown the turkey on all sides.

4. Remove the turkey from the pan using a slotted spoon. Set aside.

5. Heat the remaining oil in the same pan, and sweat the onion for about 10 minutes until soft.

6. Stir in the remaining flour and cook for 1 minute.

7. Pour in the stock, bring to the boil and simmer until thickened.

8. Return the turkey to the pan, add the ham, peas and herbs, and simmer for 5 minutes. Stir in the crème fraîche.

9. Transfer the mixture to a medium baking dish and allow to cool.

10. Lay out the puff pastry, rolling if necessary, to a size just larger than the top of the baking dish.

11. Brush the edge of the dish with a little egg and lay the pastry on top, pressing gently to seal.

12. Crimp lightly around the edges with your fingers or a fork. Brush the top of the pastry with the beaten egg. Make small slits in the top for steam to escape.

13. Bake for 30–35 minutes until the filling is completely heated through and the pastry golden brown.

14. Serve hot.

Peas Pilaf One-Pot

Ingredients:

- 7 oz tomatoes, chopped
- 5 oz green peas
- 2 fl oz Greek-style yogurt
- 4 teaspoons minced garlic
- 4 teaspoons minced root ginger
- 2 teaspoons ground coriander
- 1 teaspoon ground cumin
- 1 teaspoon garam masala
- 1/4 teaspoon ground turmeric
- 2 tablespoons canola oil
- 7 oz onion, finely diced
- 2 fresh green chillies, seeded and chopped
- 2 cinnamon sticks
- 16 black peppercorns

- 2 teaspoons cumin seeds
- 12 oz potatoes, cut into bite-sized pieces
- 7 oz basmati rice, rinsed and drained
- Salt
- freshly ground black pepper

Procedure:

1. Put the tomatoes, peas, yogurt, garlic, ginger, coriander, cumin, garam masala and turmeric in a large bowl.
2. Season with salt and pepper, and stir to combine.
3. Heat the oil in a large saucepan. Add the onion, chillies, cinnamon, peppercorns and cumin seeds, and sauté until the onion starts to turn golden.
4. Add the tomato mixture and stir through.
5. Cover and cook over a medium heat for 10 minutes, stirring occasionally.

6. Add 1,25 pt water, 3/4 teaspoon salt and the potatoes, and stir well. Cover and bring to the boil.

7. Add the rice, stir gently and cook, covered for about 10 minutes until almost all the liquid has been absorbed.

8. Reduce the heat to low, and cook for 10--15 minutes until the rice is tender.

9. Serve hot.

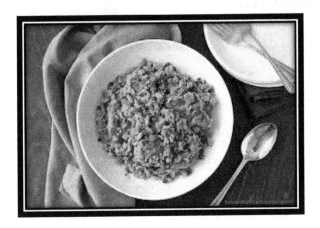

Duck, tomato & Pepper stew

<u>Serves 4</u>

Ingredients:

- 4 duck legs, each cut into 2 pieces
- 3 tablespoons olive oil
- 1 small red onion, chopped
- 3 garlic cloves, finely chopped
- 1 red pepper, seeded and cut into strips
- 1 green pepper, seeded and cut into strips
- 1,5 lb tomatoes, skinned and roughly chopped
- 2 sprigs of fresh thyme
- 1 sprig of fresh rosemary
- 1/2 oz plain chocolate, finely chopped
- salt
- freshly ground black pepper

Procedure:

1. Brown the duck legs briskly in the oil over a high heat in a wide deep frying pan. Set aside.
2. Reduce the heat and sweat the onion, garlic and peppers gently in the oil until soft.
3. Add the tomatoes, thyme, rosemary, salt and pepper and 5 fl oz water.
4. Bring to the boil, return the duck to the pan and simmer for 40 minutes.
5. Stir in the chocolate and cook for a further 5 minutes.
6. Taste, adjust the seasoning and serve hot.

Turkey Casserole

Serves 8

Ingredients:

- 3 oz butter
- 2 tablespoons plain flour
- 5 fl oz single cream
- 8 oz cooked turkey, diced
- 8 oz Cheddar cheese, grated
- 1 lb potatoes, cooked and mashed
- 8 oz dry stuffing mix
- salt
- freshly ground black pepper

Procedure:

1. Preheat the oven to 350°F.
2. Melt half the butter in a saucepan over a low heat, then stir in the flour until thoroughly mixed.
3. Slowly stir in the cream and 8 fl oz cold water.
4. Season with salt and pepper. Stir over a low heat for 5 minutes. Remove from the heat.
5. Put the turkey in a lightly greased baking dish. Pour the sauce over the turkey, then sprinkle with the cheese.
6. Spread the mashed potatoes over the cheese.
7. Melt the remaining butter and add to the stuffing mix, then sprinkle the stuffing over the potato.
8. Bake in the oven, uncovered, for 45 minutes.
9. Serve hot.

Salmon & Potato Casserole

<u>Serves 4–6</u>

Ingredients :

- 9 oz smoked salmon, flaked
- 2 lb white potatoes, thinly sliced
- 1 onion, chopped
- 1o z butter
- 2 tablespoons chopped fresh flat-leaf parsley
- 1/4 teaspoon freshly ground black pepper

Procedure:

1. Preheat the oven to 350°F.
2. Lightly grease a large casserole dish with a little vegetable oil.

3. Layer half of the salmon, potato, onion, butter, parsley and pepper in the casserole dish.

4. Repeat the layers.

5. Gently pour 3 fl oz water over the layers in the casserole dish, then cover.

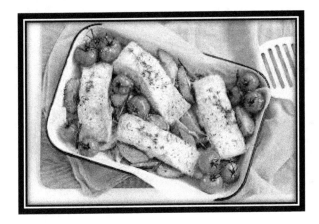

6. Bake for about 1,25 hours until the potatoes are tender.

7. Serve hot.

Prawn & Spinach Stew

<u>Serves 4</u>

Ingredients:

- 6 oz mushrooms, sliced 1 onion, chopped
- 1 garlic clove, minced
- 1 oz plain flour
- 1/8 teaspoon ground nutmeg
- 1/8 teaspoon ground black pepper
- 1 bay leaf
- 14 fl oz vegetable stock
- 8 fl oz milk
- 8 oz peeled and deveined cooked prawns
- 7 oz fresh spinach, torn
- 3 oz Gruyere cheese, grated

Procedure:

1. In a medium saucepan, cook the mushrooms, onion and garlic in the butter until soft.
2. Stir in the flour, nutmeg and pepper, and add the bay leaf.
3. Add the stock and milk, and cook, stirring, until the mixture has thickened.
4. Add the prawns and cook for a further 2 minutes.
5. Add the spinach and cheese.
6. Cook and stir until the spinach wilts and the cheese melts. Remove and discard the bay lea.
7. Serve hot.

One-Pot Cajun Chicken Gumbo

<u>Serves 2</u>

Ingredients:

- 1 tablespoon sunflower oil
- 4 chicken thighs
- 1 small onion, diced
- 2 celery sticks, diced
- 1 green pepper, seeded and diced
- 100g/4oz long-grain rice
- 300ml/10fl oz chicken stock
- 1 fresh red chilli, seeded and thinly sliced
- 225g/8oz okra, trimmed
- 1 tablespoon tomato purée salt
- freshly ground black pepper

Procedure:

1. Heat the oil in a wide pan. Fry the chicken until golden. Remove the from the pan. Stir in the onion, celery and pepper, and fry for 1 minute. Pour off any excess oil.

2. Add the rice and fry, stirring, for a further minute. Add the stock and heat until boiling. Add the chilli, okra and tomato purée. Season with salt and pepper.

3. Return the chicken to the pan and stir. Cover tightly and simmer gently for 15 minutes or until the rice is tender and the chicken is cooked. Serve immediately.

Chicken Casserole With Yogurt

Ingredients:

- 2 oz cornflour
- 1 teaspoon paprika
- 3 lb chicken fillets, skinned and trimmed
- 1 packet chicken noodle soup
- 9 fl oz warm water
- 1 garlic clove, crushed
- 1 teaspoon Worcestershire sauce
- 2 fl oz dry sherry
- 4 fl oz freshly squeezed lemon juice
- 2 tablespoons Greek-style yogurt
- 1 tablespoon finely chopped fresh flat-leaf parsley

Procedure:

1. Preheat the oven to 350°F.
2. Mix together the cornflour and paprika, and toss the chicken fillets in the mixture.
3. Arrange the fillets in the bottom of a large shallow casserole dish.
4. Combine the remaining ingredients and pour over the chicken.

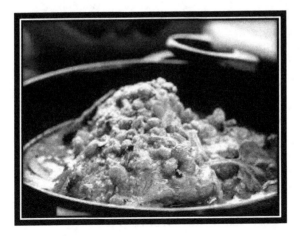

5. Cook in the oven, uncovered, for about 40 minutes until the chicken is tender.
6. Serve hot.

Squid Casserole

Ingredients:

- 3 tablespoons olive oil
- 1 large onion, thinly sliced
- 2 garlic cloves, crushed
- 1,5 lb squid rings
- 1 red pepper, seeded and sliced
- 2 sprigs of fresh rosemary
- 5 fl oz dry white wine
- 14 oz canned chopped plum tomatoes
- 2 tablespoons tomato purée
- 1 teaspoon paprika
- salt
- freshly ground black pepper

Procedure:

1. Heat the oil in a casserole dish and fry the onion and garlic until soft.
2. Add the squid, increase the heat and continue to cook for about 10 minutes until sealed and beginning to colour.
3. Add the red pepper, rosemary, wine and 9 fl oz water, and bring to the boil.
4. Cover and simmer gently for 45 minutes.
5. Discard the rosemary, and add the tomatoes, tomato purée and paprika. Season with salt and pepper.
6. Continue to simmer gently to 45–60 minutes until tender.
7. Serve hot.

Japanese Tofu Hotpot

<u>Serves 2</u>

Ingredients:

- 2 oz dried fish flakes
- 11 oz firm tofu, cubed
- 2 tablespoons light soy sauce
- 1 tablespoon granulated sugar
- 1 tablespoon sake
- 1 large egg, beaten
- 7 spring onions, roughly chopped

Procedure:

1. Spread the fish flakes evenly in the bottom of a flameproof casserole dish, and arrange the tofu on top.
2. Add the soy sauce, sugar, sake and 125ml/4fl oz water.
3. Cover and bring to the boil over a medium heat, then reduce the heat and simmer for 5 minutes.
4. Pour in the egg evenly over the top of the casserole, and sprinkle with the spring onions.
5. Simmer for a further 30 seconds, covered, then serve immediately.

Crab & Seafood One-Pot

Ingredients:

- 8 oz cooked crabmeat, shredded
- 8 oz peeled and deveined cooked prawns, chopped
- 4 fl oz sour cream
- 5 oz green chillies, sliced
- 1 teaspoon chilli powder
- 1/2 teaspoon ground cumin
- 1/4 teaspoon salt
- 8 oz tortilla chips, crushed
- 8 fl oz ready-made salsa
- 7 oz Cheddar cheese, grated
- 4 oz pitted black olives, halved
- 2 spring onions, sliced

Procedure:

1. Preheat the oven to 350°F.
2. In large bowl, mix together the crabmeat, prawns, sour cream, chillies, chilli powder, cumin and salt.

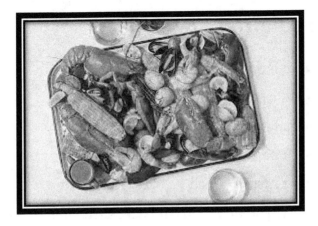

3. Line the bottom of a large baking dish with tortilla chips.
4. Spoon the crab mixture over the chips and top with salsa, cheese, olives and spring onions.
5. Bake in the oven for 15 minutes or until heated through and the cheese has melted.
6. Serve immediately.

Hearty Fish Stew

Ingredients:

- 1 large onion, thinly sliced
- 2 carrots, thinly sliced
- 1 large potato, diced
- 1 parsnip, diced
- 1 turnip, diced
- 1/4 small green cabbage, shredded
- 1 oz butter
- 14 oz canned chopped tomatoes
- 1 fish stock cube
- 12 oz cod fillet, skinned and cubed
- 12 teaspoon dried mixed herbs
- salt
- ground black pepper

Procedure:

1. Put all the vegetables in a large saucepan with the butter. Cook, stirring, for 5 minutes.
2. Add the tomatoes, 10 fl oz water and crumbled stock cube.
3. Bring to the boil, reduce the heat, part-cover and simmer for 15 minutes or until the vegetables are nearly tender.
4. Add the fish, a little salt and pepper, and the herbs, and cook for a further 5 minutes. Taste and adjust the seasoning if necessary.
5. Serve hot.

Red Snapper Casserole

<u>Serves 6</u>

Ingredients:

- 1,5 lb red snapper fillets plain flour for dredging
- 2 oz butter
- 6 oz green chilli sauce
- 12 oz Cheddar cheese, grated
- 2 tablespoons chopped fresh flat-leaf parsley
- salt
- freshly ground black pepper

Procedure:

1. Preheat the oven to 350°F.

2. Season a little flour with salt and pepper. Dredge the snapper fillets in the seasoned flour.

3. Heat the butter in a frying pan, and lightly sauté the fillets on both sides, in batches if necessary.

4. Transfer the fillets to a large casserole dish. Divide the chilli sauce and cheese among them. Bake for about 12 minutes.

5. Sprinkle with the parsley, and serve immediately.

Aromatic Green Casserole

Ingredients:

- 3 oz sugarsnap peas, cut into bite-size pieces
- 3 oz Brussels sprouts
- 3 oz broccoli, cut into bite-size pieces
- 2 oz walnuts, chopped
- 2 tablespoons vegetable oil
- 1/2 teaspoon chopped fresh dill
- 1/4 teaspoon sage
- 1/2 teaspoon salt
- juice of 1/2 lemon
- pinch of cayenne pepper

Procedure:

1. Steam the beans, Brussels sprouts and broccoli for 8 minutes.
2. Reserving the sprouts and broccoli, combine the beans with the remaining ingredients.

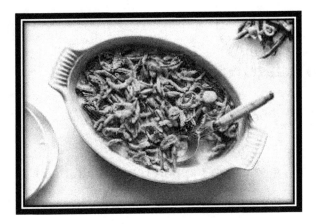

3. Transfer to a blender or food processor. Add 2 fl oz water, and purée until smooth.
4. Pour the sauce over the vegetables.
5. Serve hot or cold.

Scallop Casserole

Ingredients:

- 4 oz celery, chopped
- 4 oz onion, chopped
- 5 oz green pepper, roughly chopped
- 7 oz broccoli, chopped
- 12 oz scallops, chopped
- 3 eggs, beaten
- 7 oz Cheddar cheese, grated
- 1 teaspoon salt

Procedure:

1. Preheat the oven to 375°F.
2. In a frying pan, sauté the celery, onions and green pepper for 3–4 minutes. Cool slightly.
3. Remove from the heat and drain.
4. Cook the broccoli until tender.
5. Put the scallops and vegetables in a casserole dish. Mix gently to distribute evenly.
6. Whisk together the eggs, cheese and salt. Pour over the top of the scallops and vegetables.
7. Bake in the oven for 35–40 minutes, and serve hot.

THANK YOU!

Thank you so much for choosing my Ultimate Guide **"Quick & Easy Hotpots and Stews for Beginners"**, I've selected and cooked during my travels around the world!

To me these Stew and Hotpot Recipes are absolutely the best, with the best flavors! And, of course, they are highly recommended if you have guests for dinner!

I hope you enjoyed making the recipes as much as tasting them!

I'm already making a selection of the best Starters and Canapés for my next cookbook, so don't miss it!

CPSIA information can be obtained
at www.ICGtesting.com
Printed in the USA
BVHW090030240521
607981BV00002B/193

9 781802 997729